TO YOUR HEALTH AND BEYOND

TO YOUR HEALTH AND BEYOND

PATRICIA MILLER

"OUR DAILY BREAD"

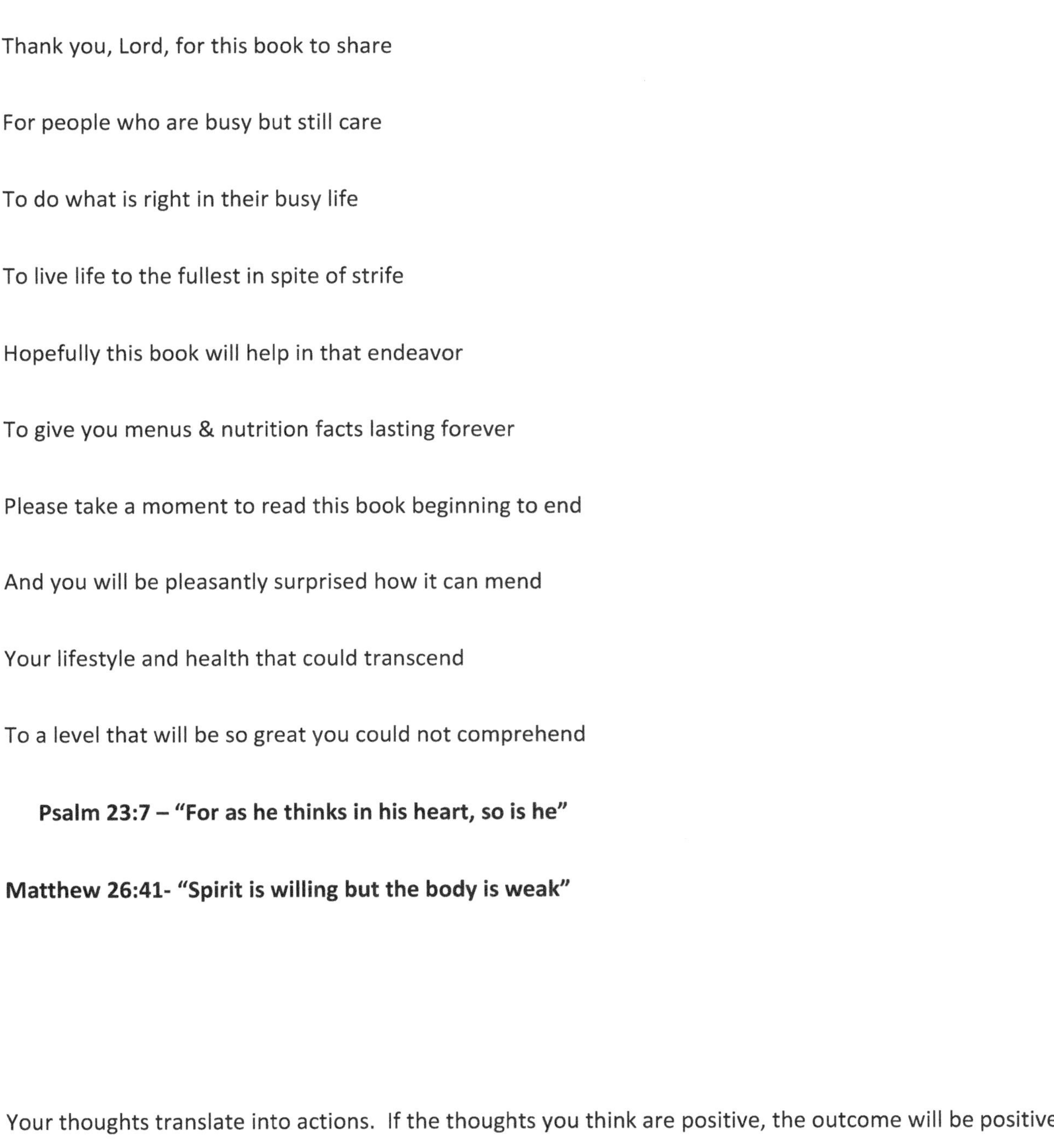

Thank you, Lord, for this book to share

For people who are busy but still care

To do what is right in their busy life

To live life to the fullest in spite of strife

Hopefully this book will help in that endeavor

To give you menus & nutrition facts lasting forever

Please take a moment to read this book beginning to end

And you will be pleasantly surprised how it can mend

Your lifestyle and health that could transcend

To a level that will be so great you could not comprehend

Psalm 23:7 – "For as he thinks in his heart, so is he"

Matthew 26:41- "Spirit is willing but the body is weak"

Your thoughts translate into actions. If the thoughts you think are positive, the outcome will be positive, if your thoughts you harbor are negative, the outcome will be negative.

<u>DEDICATION</u>

I want to express my sincere gratitude for the support & influence I received for this book from my Mom & Dad, twin sister Penny Dunovsky, my loving & very supportive husband Don and my best friend Mary Jane Foster from Parma, Ohio who has been a great support in this endeavor. I really have to give my sister Penny a whole lot of credit for her dedication and tenacious attitude to find out the secret to healthy living and a long life. Several years ago, she was diagnosed with Rheumatoid Arthritis. So far, she is doing outstanding. She was successful in raising her bone density test from osteopenia to Normal for her age. She has an excellent Nutritionist, who has been a great resource in choosing the right foods to eat.

My sister is truly amazing in that she never quits learning more and more about healthy living. They all are very inspiring people in my life. I too realize how important it is to be cognoscente of what you are eating and how the food you choose affects you. By eating Healthy I was able to get off of blood pressure medication which I had been on for several years.

My husband also was able to get off blood pressure medication by eating healthy and losing weight.

Hope this book helps all who read it to achieve a very vibrant healthy life.

CONTENTS

CHAPTER 1

VITAMINS AND MINERALS

Vitamin A

Benefits - Vitamin A is necessary for maintaining healthy tissue in the body, bone and tooth growth and night vision. Vitamin A comes directly from animal sources and is converted in the body, when necessary, from beta-carotene in plant sources.

Good Sources - Yellow or orange fruits and vegetables fortified oatmeal, liver and dairy products.

Vitamin B_1 (thiamine)

Benefits – Vitamin B_1 –Helps the body release energy from carbohydrates during metabolism; growth and muscle tone.

Good Sources – Fortified cereals and oatmeal, meats, rice and pasta, whole grains, liver.

Vitamin B_2 (riboflavin)

Benefits - Helps the body release energy from protein, fat and carbohydrates, during metabolism

Good Sources – Whole grains, green leafy vegetables, organ meats, milk and eggs.

Vitamin B_6 (pyroxidine) Helps build body tissue and aide in metabolism of protein

Good Sources – fish, poultry, lean meats, bananas, prunes, dried beans, whole grain, avocados.

Vitamin B ^{12} (cobalamin)

Benefits – Aids cell development, functioning of the nervous system and the metabolism of protein and fat.

Good Sources – Meats, milk products, seafood.

Vitamin C (ascorbic acid)

Benefits – Vitamin C is vital for the structures of bones, cartilage, muscle and blood vessels. Also helps maintain capillaries and gums, aids in the absorption of iron and may reduce the risk of some cancers.

Good Sources – Citrus fruits, berries and vegetables, especially peppers.

Vitamin D –

Benefits - Vitamin D aides in bone and tooth formation. Helps maintain hearts action and the nervous system.

Good Sources – Fortified milk, sunlight, fish, eggs, butter and fortified margarine.

Vitamin E

Benefits – Protects blood cells, body tissue and essential fatty acids from destruction in the body; may reduce the risk of coronary heart disease.

Good Sources – Fortified and multigrain cereals, nuts, wheat germ, vegetable_oils, green leafy vegetables

<u>**Vitamin K**</u>

<u>**Benefits –**</u> Necessary for blood clotting functions.

<u>**Good Sources –**</u> Green leafy vegetables, fruit, dairy and grain products.

<u>MORE NUTRITION FACTS</u>

<u>SOY</u>

"If you were to carefully review the thousands of studies published on soy, I strongly believe you would reach the same conclusion as I have-which is, the risks of consuming unfermented soy products far outweigh any possible health benefits.

Notice I said unfermented soy products.

For centuries, Asian people have been consuming fermented soy products such as natto, tempeh, and soy sauce, and enjoying the health benefits. Fermented soy does not wreak havoc on your body like unfermented soy products do. Unfortunately, many Americans who are committed to healthy lifestyles have been hoodwinked and manipulated into believing that unfermented and processed soy products like soy milk, soy cheese, soy burgers and soy ice cream are good for them. Dr. Joseph Mercola, Dr. Kaala Daniel, author of the "Whole Soy Story".

Another unfortunate fact is that 80 percent of the world's soy is used in form animal feed, which is why soy production in contributing to deforestation. Some soy propagandists have suggested that the solution to this is for all of us to become vegetarians-a reckless recommendation rooted in total ignorance amount nutrition-whereas a far better solution is a major overhaul in how farm animals are fed and raised.

FRUCTOSE/ SUGAR

Fructose also has a significant impact on triglycerides. Triglycerides are a form of fat that makes up most of your body's fat store and is also found in your blood. High levels of triglycerides in the blood have been long recognized as independent risk factor for heart disease. But in many previous human studies on fructose, researchers have measured fasting triglycerides, and fructose did not always have much effect on fasting levels. But in this study, researchers measured triglycerides after eating-what's called a post-prandial measurement. In the fructose group, post prandial triglycerides more than doubled.

It's important to remember that fructose as found in most snacks. Fruit contains small amount of fructose, but in a base of fiber and antioxidants. High fructose corn syrup is pure sweetener, with none of the benefits of fruit and baker's dozens of metabolic risks.

The American Heart Association warns that sugar may show up with other names on a label, and in higher concentrations. That is because sugary ingredients can also be listed as corn syrup, agave nectar, barley malt syrup or dehydrated can juice, just to name a few, says the source. Also keep an eye out for additives that end in "ose" like fructose.

SALT

The general rule of thumb to follow is: anything that is man-made or processed has salt in it and most of the time, it is a lot. Some of the signs of too much salt is excessive thirst, high blood pressure.

Reader's Digest presents the evidence of a 2011 Canadian study which looked at 1,200 sedentary adults who ate a high-sodium diet and found that they were at a higher risk for cognitive decline. These results were up against adults who did not eat a high sodium diet.

"Too much salt can cause blood vessels in the brain to expand, which can lead to painful headaches," she says. Women's Health.

Are you having trouble remember things or taking in information? In addition to suffering from what's called a "brain fog". People who eat too much salt will also have trouble with their memory and could increase their risk of later developing dementia or cerebrovascular diseases. WebMD cites a recent study that shows a link between high-salt diet and memory thinking problem.

The Centers for Disease Control and Prevention (CDC) estimates that the average American adult gets about 3,400 grams of sodium each day but the American Heart Association recommends the average adults should not get anymore than 1,500-milligrams per day (Yikes!)

Some of the offenders with high amounts of sodium are dome bagels, bread, deli meats, soups, Pasta sauces, pizza especially the fast varieties. However, they can be so loaded with salt that we'd be doing a disservice by not mentioning them. One particular cheeseburger from a popular fast food chain that is piled with cheese and bacon has a staggering 2860-milligrams of sodium, notes Health.com. (And that is without fries or soda!)

<u>FREQUENT URINATION</u>

Study done in Japan by Japanese doctor Dr.Matsuo Tomohroj from "When there is too

Much sodium floating around the blood, water leaves the cells, causing swelling", says Mandy Enright to Women's Health. Extreme levels of sodium, followed by excess levels of fluid to balance it out, can lead to bloating, particularly the belly area, "Nagasaki University in Japan.

Reader's Digest writes that too much salt can "increase the amount of protein found in your urine. More protein in the urine is a 'major risk factor' for kidney disease."

<u>**ARE YOU GETTING TOO MUCH SALT IN YOUR DIET? PROBABLY NOT**</u>

<u>Wall Street Journal June 2019</u>

Dietary guidelines often change, "but restrict your salt intake" has resisted the advances of science. The National Academy of Medicine has recently reiterated its' advice to limit daily intake of sodium to 2300 mg (a little over a teaspoon of salt) or 1500 mg of salt to those at risk of cardiovascular disease. An article last week in the New England Journal of Medicine indorsed that view and called for the Food and Drug Administration to impose voluntary sodium limits on 150 food categories.

These recommendations ignore scientific developments and may be harmful to your health. In March we published an article in Lancet summarizing six decades of research on sodium intake in more than a million people world-wide. We found the sodium "sweet spot"-the intake range associated with the lowest risk of disease and the longest 3,000 and 5,000 milligrams a day, considerably higher than the usual recommendations. Once daily sodium consumption falls below 3,200 milligrams, all-cause mortality increases and life expectancy decreases dramatically.

Adequate sodium is crucial for biological processes including nerve conduction, muscle contraction, and sustaining the fluid balance necessary to assure blood flow and deliver nutrients and oxygen to every cell in the body. As recently reviewed in the New England Journal of Medicine, human physiology, has evolved a complex process, mediated but the brain, to maintain sodium balance precisely. If we consume too little sodium, our kidneys will go to extremes to conserve it. If we consume too much, it is eliminated through our skin, intestines, and kidneys. You are far likelier to die from failure to maintain this precise control than from the modest impact salt may have on your blood pressure.

People listen to their bodies. Despite vigorous efforts by government and advocacy groups, average U.S. sodium intake has remained constant at 3,600 to 3,700 milligrams a day. In 2005 the British government undertook a determined effort to reduce sodium content in processed food, as the FDA is now being urged to. Britons adjusted their eating habits. In 2014 the government reported that the reductions in sodium content had led to no significant change in sodium intake.

Understanding the stark contrast between the National Academy of Medicine's recommendations and what science has identified as sodium's healthy range is critical to the nation's health. Minimal decreases in serum sodium predict increased mortality in healthy people. Although this is not fully understood, we know that risk increases when sodium intake breeches the lower limits of the brain's ability to maintain serum sodium within its narrow range-especially in healthy middle-aged men, for whom it nearly doubles the risks. Comparable increases in risk exist for the ill and the elderly. Low serum sodium at hospital admission is associated with increased length of stay, in hospital death, and discharge to a care facility. If contrary to the British experience, the prospective FDA restrictions on sodium in food prove successful in reducing intake that could magnify the risk for Americans.

The U.S. department of Agriculture and the Health and Human Services Department are currently deliberating their quinquennial federal dietary guidelines, with release lasted for next year. The government should address and incorporate all available evidence into its dietary guidance. Fortunately, no government policy can override our craving for salt.

<u>**GOOD NEWS FOR CARB LOVERS**</u>

<u>Consumer Report Magazine (March) 2019</u>

Good news for carb lovers: There reason not to shun carbohydrate-even some of you may not think of as healthy.

That is because certain foods provide what's called resistant starch, or RS, which offers some of fiber's benefits.

Resistant starch lowers blood sugar after a meal, helps reduce appetite, is M.D. an assistant professor medicine at Hofstra Northwell School of Medicine in New York.

<u>HOW RESISTANT STARCH HELPS YOU</u>

One key action of resistant starch is that it helps keep your microbial balance healthy, providing a greater proportion of "good" to "bad" gut bacteria.

How? When you eat resistant starch, it passes undigested through the small intestine-where-nutrients are absorbed-to the colon. There, it fuels the body's good bacteria.

And those healthy gut microbes, says Kane, play a role in almost every organ system in the body, including the gastrointestinal and immune.

"If you don't get enough fermentable fiber, like resistant starch, you risk the buildup of mucus-consuming bacteria that will degrade the protective lining of your intestines, allowing pathogens to gain access", explains Michael Keenan, Ph.D., a professor of nutrition and food sciences at Louisiana State University.

A thinner-than-optimal mucus layer might make you more susceptible to inflammatory bowel disease and colon cancer, for example.

In addition, blood sugar (glucose) levels rise more slowly after meals with resistant starch, which helps the body better use hormone insulin. This may improve type 2 diabetes control and weight management.

The starch might even increase fat burning. According to a small study published in the journal Nutrition & Metabolism, people burned 23 percent more fat after a meal with 5 percent resistant starch than they usually did after a meal without it.

<u>WHERE TO GET RESISTANT STARCH</u>

One type of resistant starch-there are five types-is found in whole grains and seeds, another in certain legumes (chickpeas, kidney beans, lentils) and under ripe bananas.

In fact green bananas are the best source of resistant starch. (The starch turns to sugars as the fruit ripens.)

Unprocessed foods are generally the healthiest way to get resistant starch, but there are exceptions. Pasta, potatoes, and the white rice are good sources of the type of resistant starch that forms when foods are cooked, then cooled-a process that alters the chemical structure of the carbs in these foods.

Eating them cold or at room temperature can be appetizing too: Think pasta or potato salad.

How much resistant starch should you get? You need to consume 25 to 30 grams of fiber per day, but there is no such recommendation for resistant starch.

"We do not really know how much we need because we do not even really know how to measure it properly," says Diand Birt, PhD. distinguished professor of food science and human nutrition at Iowa State University.

The best way to get enough to reap its benefits is to increase your fiber intake, and to eat foods that contain it.

What about resistant starch supplements (notable from potato starch)? "It's hard to get too much of a nutrient when you get it in food", Birt says. "But with supplements we don't know how much is too much, and they may interfere with absorption and bioavailability or other nutrients.

And when you get resistant starch from foods, you get many at the other fiber in foods works along with resistant starch in beneficial ways.

Author

Martica Heaner, PhD.

Martica Heaner is an adjunct associate nutrition professor at Hunter College in NYC and in exercise physiologist. She has been a health writer for 30 years and is the author of eight books on health and fitness. She has written for the New York Time, The Time London, Glenour, Shape, Men's Health, Family Circle, GQ, Self and other publications.

"It's summer, the season when protein-rich burgers and steaks are sizzling on outdoor grills. That got us wondering: How much protein should an adult consume every day? Most dieticians consider these nutrients a building block of a healthy diet. Proteins, which are long chains of amino acids, are the basic components of tissue found in all human muscles and internal organs.

Janell Walter, a professor of family and consumer sciences at Baylor University in Waco Texas, served up dome advice on protein sources, portion sizes, fad diets and a powerful pairing for vegetarians.

THE GOLDEN NUTRIENT

Unlike carbohydrates or fats, proteins are the only nutrients that can be used to build new cells that can form tissue, said Dr. Walter, a registered dietician. Our bodies, thanks especially to our livers, are "protein-making machines," she said, but among the 22 amino acids found in proteins, nine cannot be made by the body. These have to be supplied by food, and the best source of them is what we call a complete protein, which included meat, chicken, fish, milk or eggs," she said, and the type of complete protein it comes from doesn't matter in a balanced diet that included fruits, vegetables and grains.

Though plant proteins found in nuts, tofu, chickpeas and other sources do contain amino acids, none have all of those nine essential ones on their own, However, Professor Walter said, there is magical combination: If you put a nut or legume with a grain product, they complement each other to give the body what it needs". But it takes one and a half cups of rice and beans to equal the protein in three ounces of meat. "You have to eat a heck of a lot of food if you get you protein from plants versus animal products," Dr. Walter said. Meat is just more efficient". A gram of meat has the same number of calories as a gram of carbohydrates, she said.

<u>IRON AND ZINC</u>

Two meat patties, the size of the palm of an average adult's hand, are the right amount of protein to eat a day. Whether fresh, frozen, grilled or even canned, any animal protein retains its nutritional value. "Protein doesn't get destroyed or inactivated with cooking, freezing or processing," Dr. Walter said. In a restaurant, an "18 oz. steak" probably includes the bone, fat and gristle before cooking, so the true serving is about 13 ounces-still more than one adult require a day

Although at least one study has shown that eating grilled meat can cause cancer, "you would have to eat lots and lots of charred meat for long time to get enough carcinogens to have a negative effect, "Dr. Walter said. She is a big fan of shrimp but eats all forms of animal proteins. She cooks meat thoroughly to avoid natural occurring bacteria such as E. coli and salmonella. Also "the body can break down protein a little bit better when it's cooked, "she adds.

Unlike fish, light-colored meat or plant foods, only red meat has the ideal balance of iron and zinc, which the body requires to be taken together in order to, be absorbed by the digestive tract. "You can supplement your diet to get the right balance, but you should do it with a dietician," the professor said. Too much iron or zinc can cause abdominal or worse, she said. Dr. Walter also said that, despite pervasive myths, "Serving per serving of lean red meat has no more cholesterol than any other land animal".

Dr. Walter sometimes refers patients to the USDA's meal-planning site, choosemyplate.gov, which has diet plans based on age and activity level. "For some reason, every drink and meal replacement bar claim it has extra protein-which we don't need" she said. "People see protein as a magical nutrient with no side effects, which is way off-target—and protein is not cheap".

OVERDOING IT

Cooked red meat is the most efficient source for of protein, but if you eat more than eight ounces a day, it will be stored as fat, said Dr. Walter, "though the American carnivorous diet typically has more than enough protein than adults need." In countries without enough meat, she added, adolescent's growth often is stunted, which can't be reversed. "In additions, their internal organs developed during that period may have fewer cells, which can cause problems much later in life," she said.

For grownups, a phase of protein deficiency can lead to anemia, tissue not healing as quickly as normal and difficulty fighting off infections. But all those can be addressed quickly by balancing one's eating. Dr. Walter said. She takes tissue with fad diets that restrict carbohydrates in favor of proteins, because the brain runs in carbs and eliminating them can lead to dehydration. In addition, laying on the protein can tax the liver. "People love to lose weight, but they often don't care where the pounds come from" she lamented. "

MENUS IN TABLE FORM

Saturday 3/4/17 **Hamburgers** **Saturday 3/11/17** *Steak*	***Sunday 3/5/17*** ***Pork Roast*** ***Sunday 3/12/17*** ***Chicken Roast***
Monday 3/6/17 **Leftovers** ***Monday 3/13/17*** **Leftovers**	***Tuesday 3/7/17*** ***Southwestern Hash*** ***Tuesday 3/14/17*** ***Sausage grilled/boiled***
Wednesday 3/8/17 *Meatballs* *Wednesday 3/15/17* *Pizza*	*Thursday 3/9/17* *Lamb chops* *Thursday 3/16/17* **Sweet & Sour Pork**
Friday 3/10/17 **Fish – Lent Salmon** ***Friday 3/17/17*** *Eat out*	**Tomato Soup** **Tuna Salad** **Lamb Chops**

<u>BREADS, PASTAS, POTATOES</u>
Wheat Bread
English muffins
No Yolk Noodles
Spiral Pasta
5 lbs. Red potatoes

<u>DAIRY PRODUCTS</u>
Butter
Sour cream
Almond Milk
Cream cheese
2% cheddar cheese brick
Add new items -

<u>VEGETABLES</u>
Celery
Zucchini
Cucumber
Tomatoes
Add new items -

<u>MEATS</u>
Grass Fed Beef
Pork Chops
Chicken thighs
Chicken breasts
Bacon
Add new items -

<u>CLEANING PRODUCTS</u>
Dishwasher soap
Floor cleaner
Cleaning sponges
Toilet Bowl cleaner
Add new items -

<u>**CANNED GOODS**</u>
Canned corn
Black beans
Green beans
Tomato sauce
Spaghetti sauce
Add new items –

<u>**FROZEN FOODS**</u>
Vegetables
Desserts

<u>**MISCELLANEOUS**</u>
Hair spray
Deodorant
Shoe polish
Light bulbs
Air filters
Add new items -

Saturday 3/18/17 **Beefy stuffed zucchini/sausage** **_Saturday 3/25/17_** **_Steak_**	**_Sunday 3/19/17_** **_Beef Roast_** **_Sunday 3/26/17_** **_Cauliflower soup_**
Monday 3/20/17 **Leftovers** **_Monday 3/27/17_** **Leftovers**	**_Tuesday 3/21/17_** **Tomato Soup** **_Tuesday 3/28/17_** **Pea Soup**
Wednesday 3/22/17 **Hamburgers** **_Wednesday 3/29/17_** **Leftovers**	**_Thursday 3/23/17_** **Lamb chops** **_Thursday 3/30/17_** **Almond pancakes/sausage links**
Friday 3/24/17 **_Fish – Lent Scallops/Shrimp_** **_Friday 3/31/17_** _Eat out_	**_Grilled Vegetables_** **_Cornish Hen_** **_Stuffed Zucchini_** **_Stuffed green peppers_**

<u>**BREADS, PASTAS, POTATOES**</u>
Wheat Bread
English muffins
No Yolk Noodles
Spiral Pasta
5 lbs. Red potatoes

<u>**DAIRY PRODUCTS**</u>
Butter
Sour cream
Almond Milk
Cream cheese
2% cheddar cheese brick
Add new items -

<u>**VEGETABLES**</u>
Celery
Zucchini
Cucumber
Tomatoes
Add new items -

<u>**MEATS**</u>
Grass Fed Beef
Pork Chops
Chicken thighs
Chicken breasts
Bacon
Add new items -

<u>**CLEANING PRODUCTS**</u>
Dishwasher soap
Floor cleaner
Cleaning sponges
Toilet Bowl cleaner
Add new items -

<u>CANNED GOODS</u>
Canned corn
Black beans
Green beans
Tomato sauce
Spaghetti sauce
Add new items –

<u>FROZEN FOODS</u>
Vegetables
Desserts

<u>MISCELLANEOUS</u>
Hair spray
Deodorant
Shoe polish
Light bulbs
Air filters
Add new items -

Saturday 4/27/19 **Come back from Statesville -Pizza** *Saturday 5/4/19* *Lamb chops*	*Sunday 4/28/19* **Chicken Roast** *Sunday 5/5/19* *Standing rib roast*
Monday 4/29/19 *Leftovers* *Monday 5/6/19* *Leftovers*	*Tuesday 4/30/19* *Spaghetti/sausage* *Tuesday 5/7/19* *Leave for Cleveland*
Wednesday 5/1/19 *Chili* *Wednesday 5/8/19* *Sausage*	*Thursday 5/2/19* *Leftovers* *Thursday 5/9/19* **Shake & bake chicken**
Friday 5/3/19 *Homestyle gumbo –p.77 Healthy* *Homestyle meals* *Friday 5/10/19* *Mediterranean chicken sauté stir fry* *P.39 stir fry*	

<u>BREADS, PASTAS, POTATOES</u>
Wheat Bread
English muffins
No Yolk Noodles
Spiral Pasta
5 lbs. Red potatoes

<u>DAIRY PRODUCTS</u>
Butter
Sour cream
Almond Milk
Cream cheese
2% cheddar cheese brick
Add new items -

<u>VEGETABLES</u>
Celery
Zucchini
Cucumber
Tomatoes
Add new items -

<u>MEATS</u>
Grass Fed Beef
Pork Chops
Chicken thighs
Chicken breasts
Bacon
Add new items -

<u>CLEANING PRODUCTS</u>
Dishwasher soap
Floor cleaner
Cleaning sponges
Toilet Bowl cleaner
Add new items -

<u>CANNED GOODS</u>
Canned corn
Black beans
Green beans
Tomato sauce
Spaghetti sauce
Add new items –

<u>FROZEN FOODS</u>
Vegetables
Desserts

<u>MISCELLANEOUS</u>
Hair spray
Deodorant
Shoe polish
Light bulbs
Air filters
Add new items -

Saturday 4/13/19 **Steak** _Saturday 4/20/19_ _Lamb chops_	_Sunday 4/14/19_ **Pork Roast** _Sunday 4/21/19_ _EASTER_
Monday 4/15/19 _Leftovers_ _Monday 4/22/19_ _Leftovers_	_Tuesday 4/16/19_ _Meatloaf_ _Tuesday 4/23/19_ _Pizza_
Wednesday 4/17/19 _Southwestern zucchini boats P.34_ _Quick cooking_ _Wednesday 4/24/19_ _Sweet & Sauerkraut bratwurst sandwich p57 Lazy Day cooking_	_Thursday 4/18/19_ _Sausage_ _Thursday 4/25/19_ **Leftover turkey a la king**
Friday 4/19/19 _Shrimp & vegetable stir fry p.17 chicken &fish_ _Friday 4/26/19_ _Tuna noodle casserole-steak_	**Homestyle gumbo –p.77 Healthy Homestyle meals** **Spaghetti/sausage** **Mediterranean chicken sauté stir fry P.39 stir fry**

<u>**BREADS, PASTAS, POTATOES**</u>
Wheat Bread
English muffins
No Yolk Noodles
Spiral Pasta
5 lbs. Red potatoes

<u>**DAIRY PRODUCTS**</u>
Butter
Sour cream
Almond Milk
Cream cheese
2% cheddar cheese brick
Add new items -

<u>**VEGETABLES**</u>
Celery
Zucchini
Cucumber
Tomatoes
Add new items -

<u>**MEATS**</u>
Grass Fed Beef
Pork Chops
Chicken thighs
Chicken breasts
Bacon
Add new items -

<u>**CLEANING PRODUCTS**</u>
Dishwasher soap
Floor cleaner
Cleaning sponges
Toilet Bowl cleaner
Add new items -

<u>CANNED GOODS</u>
Canned corn
Black beans
Green beans
Tomato sauce
Spaghetti sauce
Add new items –

<u>FROZEN FOODS</u>
Vegetables
Desserts

<u>MISCELLANEOUS</u>
Hair spray
Deodorant
Shoe polish
Light bulbs
Air filters
Add new items -

Saturday 5/25/19 **Hamburgers** *Saturday 6/1/19* **Steak**	*Sunday 5/26/19* **Pork Roast** *Sunday 6/2/19* **Moroccan lentil stew p31Good for you**
Monday 5/27/19 **Leftovers** *Monday 6/3/19* **Leftovers**	*Tuesday 5/28/19* **Sweet & Sauerkraut bratwurst sandwich p57 Lazy Day cooking** *Tuesday 6/4/19* **Spaghetti/sausage**
Wednesday 5/29/19 **Hearty Spinach & Mushroom soup** *Wednesday 6/5/19* **Sausage**	*Thursday 5/30/19* **Cabbage, potato & sausage soup** *Thursday 6/6/19* **Lamb chops**
Friday 5/31/19 **Eggs sausage, green pepper, potatoes** *Friday 6/7/19* **Imitation crab salad**	**Crab cakes** **shrimp**

<u>BREADS, PASTAS, POTATOES</u>
Wheat Bread
English muffins
No Yolk Noodles
Spiral Pasta
5 lbs. Red potatoes

<u>DAIRY PRODUCTS</u>
Butter
Sour cream
Almond Milk
Cream cheese
2% cheddar cheese brick
Add new items -

<u>VEGETABLES</u>
Celery
Zucchini
Cucumber
Tomatoes
Add new items -

<u>MEATS</u>
Grass Fed Beef
Pork Chops
Chicken thighs
Chicken breasts
Bacon
Add new items -

<u>CLEANING PRODUCTS</u>
Dishwasher soap
Floor cleaner
Cleaning sponges
Toilet Bowl cleaner
Add new items -

<u>**CANNED GOODS**</u>
Canned corn
Black beans
Green beans
Tomato sauce
Spaghetti sauce
Add new items –

<u>**FROZEN FOODS**</u>
Vegetables
Desserts

<u>**MISCELLANEOUS**</u>
Hair spray
Deodorant
Shoe polish
Light bulbs
Air filters
Add new items -

Saturday 6/8/19 *steak* *Saturday 6/15/19* *Shake & Bake chicken*	*Sunday 6/9/19* *Chicken Roast* *Sunday 6/16/19* *Stuffed peppers*
Monday 6/10/19 *Leftovers* *Monday 6/17/19* *Leftovers*	*Tuesday 6/11/19* *Sweet & Sauerkraut bratwurst sandwich p57 Lazy Day cooking* *Tuesday 6/18/19* *Spaghetti/sausage*
Wednesday 6/12/19 *Eat Out* *Wednesday 6/19/19* *Sausage*	*Thursday 6/13/19* *Cabbage, potato & sausage soup* *Thursday 6/20/19* *Lamb chops*
Friday 6/14/19 *Eggs sausage, green pepper, potatoes* *Friday 6/21/19* *Imitation crab salad*	*Crab cakes* *Shrimp* *Meatloaf* *Vegetarian lasagna*

BREADS, PASTAS, POTATOES
Wheat Bread
English muffins
No Yolk Noodles
Spiral Pasta
5 lbs. Red potatoes

DAIRY PRODUCTS
Butter
Sour cream
Almond Milk
Cream cheese
2% cheddar cheese brick
Add new items -

VEGETABLES
Celery
Zucchini
Cucumber
Tomatoes
Add new items -

MEATS
Grass Fed Beef
Pork Chops
Chicken thighs
Chicken breasts
Bacon
Add new items -

CLEANING PRODUCTS
Dishwasher soap
Floor cleaner
Cleaning sponges
Toilet Bowl cleaner
Add new items -

<u>CANNED GOODS</u>
Canned corn
Black beans
Green beans
Tomato sauce
Spaghetti sauce
Add new items –

<u>FROZEN FOODS</u>
Vegetables
Desserts

<u>MISCELLANEOUS</u>
Hair spray
Deodorant
Shoe polish
Light bulbs
Air filters
Add new items -

Saturday 6/22/19 steak *Saturday 6/29/19* Cornish hen	*Sunday 6/23/19* Vegetarian Lasagna *Sunday 6/30/19* Pot roast
Monday 6/24/19 Leftovers *Monday 7/1/19* Leftovers	*Tuesday 6/25/19* Meatloaf *Tuesday 7/2/19* Vegetarian supper dish
Wednesday 6/26/19 Pizza *Wednesday 7/3/19* Mediterranean chicken sauté p39stir fries	*Thursday 6/27/19* Cabbage, potato & sausage soup *Thursday 7/4/19* Fourth of July
Friday 6/28/19 Crab cakes *Friday 7/5/19* Shrimp stir fry	Shrimp Hamburgers

BREADS, PASTAS, POTATOES
Wheat Bread
English muffins
No Yolk Noodles
Spiral Pasta
5 lbs. Red potatoes

DAIRY PRODUCTS
Butter
Sour cream
Almond Milk
Cream cheese
2% cheddar cheese brick
Add new items -

VEGETABLES
Celery
Zucchini
Cucumber
Tomatoes
Add new items -

MEATS
Grass Fed Beef
Pork Chops
Chicken thighs
Chicken breasts
Bacon
Add new items -

<u>**CLEANING PRODUCTS**</u>
Dishwasher soap
Floor cleaner
Cleaning sponges
Toilet Bowl cleaner
Add new items -

<u>**CANNED GOODS**</u>
Canned corn
Black beans
Green beans
Tomato sauce
Spaghetti sauce
Add new items –

<u>**FROZEN FOODS**</u>
Vegetables
Desserts

<u>**MISCELLANEOUS**</u>
Hair spray
Deodorant
Shoe polish
Light bulbs
Air filters
Add new items -

Saturday 7/6/19 *Hamburgers* *Saturday 7/13/19* *steak*	*Sunday 7/7/19* *Chicken Roast* *Sunday 7/14/19* *Pea Soup*
Monday 7/8/19 *Leftovers* *Monday 7/15/19* *Leftovers*	*Tuesday 7/9/19* *Pizza* *Tuesday 7/16/19* *Scrambled eggs stir fry*
Wednesday 7/10/19 *Fresh Mushroom Soup* *Wednesday 7/1719* *Cornish Hen*	*Thursday 7/11/19* *sausage* *Thursday 7/18/19* *Lamb chops*
Friday 7/19/19 *Crab cakes* *Friday 7/17/19* *Shrimp*	*Scrambled eggs/ham* *Pork chops* *Spaghetti* *Autumn skillet supper p.16* *hamburger*

BREADS, PASTAS, POTATOES
Wheat Bread
English muffins
No Yolk Noodles
Spiral Pasta
5 lbs. Red potatoes

DAIRY PRODUCTS
Butter
Sour cream
Almond Milk
Cream cheese
2% cheddar cheese brick
Add new items -

VEGETABLES
Celery
Zucchini
Cucumber
Tomatoes
Add new items -

MEATS
Grass Fed Beef
Pork Chops
Chicken thighs
Chicken breasts
Bacon
Add new items -

CLEANING PRODUCTS
Dishwasher soap
Floor cleaner
Cleaning sponges
Toilet Bowl cleaner
Add new items -

<u>CANNED GOODS</u>
Canned corn
Black beans
Green beans
Tomato sauce
Spaghetti sauce
Add new items –

<u>FROZEN FOODS</u>
Vegetables
Desserts

<u>MISCELLANEOUS</u>
Hair spray
Deodorant
Shoe polish
Light bulbs
Air filters
Add new items -

Saturday 5/11/19	Sunday 5/12/19
Graduation Neighbor	Pork Roast
Saturday 5/18/19	**Sunday 5/19/19**
Cornish Hen	Newcomers thank you dinner
Monday 5/13/19	**Tuesday 5/14/19**
Leftovers	Don's Birthday
Monday 5/20/19	**Tuesday 5/21/19**
Roasted grilled vegetables	Spaghetti/sausage
Wednesday 5/15/19	**Thursday 5/16/19**
Vegetarian supper dish	Cabbage, potato & sausage soup
Wednesday 5/22/19	**Thursday 5/23/19**
Sausage	Honey Dijon pork chops
Friday 5/17/19	Hamburgers
Homestyle gumbo	Steak
	Sweet & Sauerkraut bratwurst
Friday 5/24/19	sandwich p57 Lazy Day cooking
Tuna noodle casserole	

<u>BREADS, PASTAS, POTATOES</u>
Wheat Bread
English muffins
No Yolk Noodles
Spiral Pasta
5 lbs. Red potatoes

<u>DAIRY PRODUCTS</u>
Butter
Sour cream
Almond Milk
Cream cheese
2% cheddar cheese brick
Add new items -

<u>VEGETABLES</u>
Celery
Zucchini
Cucumber
Tomatoes
Add new items -

<u>MEATS</u>
Grass Fed Beef
Pork Chops
Chicken thighs
Chicken breasts
Bacon
Add new items -

<u>CLEANING PRODUCTS</u>
Dishwasher soap
Floor cleaner
Cleaning sponges
Toilet Bowl cleaner
Add new items -

<u>**CANNED GOODS**</u>
Canned corn
Black beans
Green beans
Tomato sauce
Spaghetti sauce
Add new items –

<u>**FROZEN FOODS**</u>
Vegetables
Desserts

<u>**MISCELLANEOUS**</u>
Hair spray
Deodorant
Shoe polish
Light bulbs
Air filters
Add new items -

Saturday 7/20/19 sausage ***Saturday 7/27/19*** Hamburgers	***Sunday 7/21/19*** **Chicken noodle soup** ***Sunday 7/28/19*** **Chicken roast**
Monday 7/22/19 **Leftovers** ***Monday 7/29/19*** **Leftovers**	***Tuesday 7/23/19*** **Tuna Fish cakes** ***Tuesday 7/30/19*** **chili**
Wednesday 7/24/19 **Vegetarian supper dish** ***Wednesday 7/31/19*** **leftovers**	***Thursday 7/25/19*** **Shake & bake chicken** ***Thursday 8/1/19*** **Lamb chops**
Friday 7/26/19 **Crab cakes** ***Friday 8/2/19*** Shrimp w/sides	**Scrambled eggs/ham** **Pork chops**

<u>**BREADS, PASTAS, POTATOES**</u>
Wheat Bread
English muffins
No Yolk Noodles
Spiral Pasta
5 lbs. Red potatoes

<u>**DAIRY PRODUCTS**</u>
Butter
Sour cream
Almond Milk
Cream cheese
2% cheddar cheese brick
Add new items -

<u>**VEGETABLES**</u>
Celery
Zucchini
Cucumber
Tomatoes
Add new items -

<u>**MEATS**</u>
Grass Fed Beef
Pork Chops
Chicken thighs
Chicken breasts
Bacon
Add new items -

<u>**CLEANING PRODUCTS**</u>
Dishwasher soap
Floor cleaner
Cleaning sponges
Toilet Bowl cleaner
Add new items -

<u>CANNED GOODS</u>
Canned corn
Black beans
Green beans
Tomato sauce
Spaghetti sauce
Add new items –

<u>FROZEN FOODS</u>
Vegetables
Desserts

<u>MISCELLANEOUS</u>
Hair spray
Deodorant
Shoe polish
Light bulbs
Air filters
Add new items -

Saturday 8/3/19 **_Autumn skillet supper p.16_** **_hamburger_** **_Saturday 8/10/19_**	**_Sunday 8/4/19_** **_Chicken noodle soup_** **_Sunday 8/11/19_** **_Pork Roast_**
Monday 8/5/19 **_Leftovers_** **_Monday 8/12/19_** **_Leftovers_**	**_Tuesday 8/6/19_** **_Tuna Salad over toasted English muffins_** **_Tuesday 8/13/19_** **_Scrambled eggs/ham_**
Wednesday 8/7/19 **_Vegetarian supper dish_** **_Wednesday 8/14/19_** **_Spaghetti/sausage_**	**_Thursday 8/8/19_** **_Caesar Pork chops p.15easy weekend meals_** **_Thursday 8/15/19_** **_Lamb chops_**
Friday 8/9/19 **_Crab cakes_** **_Friday 8/16/19_** **_salmon_**	**_Spaghetti Squash_** **_2 rib eye steaks_** **_2 Cornish hens_** **_Split pea soup_**

<u>BREADS, PASTAS, POTATOES</u>
Wheat Bread
English muffins
No Yolk Noodles
Spiral Pasta
5 lbs. Red potatoes

<u>DAIRY PRODUCTS</u>
Butter
Sour cream
Almond Milk
Cream cheese
2% cheddar cheese brick
Add new items -

<u>VEGETABLES</u>
Celery
Zucchini
Cucumber
Tomatoes
Add new items -

<u>MEATS</u>
Grass Fed Beef
Pork Chops
Chicken thighs
Chicken breasts
Bacon
Add new items -

<u>CLEANING PRODUCTS</u>
Dishwasher soap
Floor cleaner
Cleaning sponges
Toilet Bowl cleaner
Add new items -

<u>CANNED GOODS</u>
Canned corn
Black beans
Green beans
Tomato sauce
Spaghetti sauce
Add new items –

<u>FROZEN FOODS</u>
Vegetables
Desserts

<u>MISCELLANEOUS</u>
Hair spray
Deodorant
Shoe polish
Light bulbs
Air filters
Add new items -

Saturday 11/23/19 *Steak* ***Saturday 11/30/19*** *Pork chops*	***Sunday 11/24/19*** *Pork Roast* ***Sunday 12/1/19*** *Stuffed peppers*
Monday 11/25/19 *Leftovers* ***Monday 12/2/19*** *Leftovers*	***Tuesday 11/26/19*** *Beans over rice* ***Tuesday 12/3/19*** *Shake & bake chicken*
Wednesday 11/27/19 *Spaghetti/sausage* ***Wednesday 12/4/19*** *Yum Yum*	***Thursday 11/28/19*** *Thanksgiving Nick & Rosemary* ***Thursday 12/5/19*** *Lamb chops*
Friday 11/29/19 *Crab cakes* ***Friday 12/6/19*** *Salmon*	*Steak* *Broccoli, spinach* *Tuna noodle casserole* *Meat loaf*

<u>**BREADS, PASTAS, POTATOES**</u>
Wheat Bread
English muffins
No Yolk Noodles
Spiral Pasta
5 lbs. Red potatoes

<u>**DAIRY PRODUCTS**</u>
Butter
Sour cream
Almond Milk
Cream cheese
2% cheddar cheese brick
Add new items -

<u>**VEGETABLES**</u>
Celery
Zucchini
Cucumber
Tomatoes
Add new items -

<u>**MEATS**</u>
Grass Fed Beef
Pork Chops
Chicken thighs
Chicken breasts
Bacon
Add new items -

CLEANING PRODUCTS
Dishwasher soap
Floor cleaner
Cleaning sponges
Toilet Bowl cleaner
Add new items -

CANNED GOODS
Canned corn
Black beans
Green beans
Tomato sauce
Spaghetti sauce
Add new items –

FROZEN FOODS
Vegetables
Desserts

MISCELLANEOUS
Hair spray
Deodorant
Shoe polish
Light bulbs
Air filters

<table>
<tr><td>

Saturday 12/7/19
Steak

Saturday 12/16/19
Pork chops

</td><td>

Sunday 12/8/19
Pork Roast

Sunday 12/17/19
Turkey

</td></tr>
<tr><td>

Monday 12/9/19
Leftovers

Monday 12/18/19
Leftovers

</td><td>

Tuesday 12/10/19
Chili

Tuesday 12/19/19
Sausage

</td></tr>
<tr><td>

Wednesday 12/11/19
Leftover chili

Wednesday 12/20/19
Spinach & Mushroom Soup

</td><td>

Thursday 12/12/19
Turkey & peas casserole

Thursday 12/21/19
Lamb chops

</td></tr>
<tr><td>

Friday 12/15/19
Crab cakes

Friday   12/22/19
Salmon

</td><td>

Steak
Broccoli, spinach
Tuna noodle casserole
Meat loaf

</td></tr>
</table>

<u>BREADS, PASTAS, POTATOES</u>
Wheat Bread
English muffins
No Yolk Noodles
Spiral Pasta
5 lbs. Red potatoes

<u>DAIRY PRODUCTS</u>
Butter
Sour cream
Almond Milk
Cream cheese
2% cheddar cheese brick
Add new items -

<u>VEGETABLES</u>
Celery
Zucchini
Cucumber
Tomatoes
Add new items -

<u>MEATS</u>
Grass Fed Beef
Pork Chops
Chicken thighs
Chicken breasts
Bacon
Add new items -

<u>CLEANING PRODUCTS</u>
Dishwasher soap
Floor cleaner
Cleaning sponges
Toilet Bowl cleaner
Add new items -

<u>**CANNED GOODS**</u>
Canned corn
Black beans
Green beans
Tomato sauce
Spaghetti sauce
Add new items –

<u>**FROZEN FOODS**</u>
Vegetables
Desserts

<u>**MISCELLANEOUS**</u>
Hair spray
Deodorant
Shoe polish
Light bulbs
Air filters
Add new items -

CHAPTER 2

Recipes

<u>AUTUMN SKILLET SUPPER</u>

<u>1 lb. grass fed beef</u>

<u>2 cups diced eggplant</u>

<u>½ cup chopped green bell pepper</u>

<u>2 medium tomatoes chopped</u>

<u>1 garlic clove minced</u>

<u>1 (14oz) can low sodium, beef broth</u>

<u>2 cups of Basmati rice</u>

<u>1 oz. (1/4 cup) finely shredded fresh parmesan cheese</u>

<u>2 tablespoons of chopped fresh basil</u>

1. <u>Brown ground beef in large skillet over medium-high heat until thoroughly cooked, stirring frequently. Drain.</u>
2. <u>Stir in eggplant, bell pepper, tomatoes, garlic and broth. Bring to a boil. Cover simmer 5 to 6 minutes or until vegetables are tender.</u>
3. <u>Stir in cooked rice. Cover, remove from heat. Let stand 5 minutes. Fluff with fork.</u>
4. <u>Stir in cheese and basil.</u>

<u>Total carbohydrates 37g, Dietary fiber 2 g, Protein 23g, Vitamin A 10%, Calcium 20%, Vitamin C 20%, Iron 20%</u>

BUTTERNUT SQUASH

¼ teaspoon salt

18 teaspoon ground cinnamon

1/8 teaspoon ground nutmeg

1/8 teaspoon ground pepper

1 small butternut squash (about 2 lbs.)

2 tablespoon butter, melted

6 teaspoons brown sugar, divided

1. Preheat oven to 350 degrees. Mix seasoning ingredients. Halve squash lengthwise: remove and discard seeds. Place squash in an 11x7 inch baking dish coated with cooking spray. Brush with melted butter; sprinkle with seasoning.
2. Place 2 teaspoons brown sugar in the cavity of each half. Sprinkle remaining brown sugar over cut surfaces.
3. Bake, covered 40 minutes. Uncover, bake until squash is tender, about 20 minutes.

Serves 2

BALSAMIC GRILLED ZUCCHINI

2 zucchinis, quartered lengthwise

2 teaspoons olive oil

1//2 teaspoon garlic powder

1 teaspoon Italian seasoning

1 pinch salt

2 tablespoons balsamic vinegar

Add all ingredients

1. **Preheat grill for medium-low heat and lightly oil the grate.**
2. **Brush zucchini with olive oil. Sprinkle garlic powder, Italian seasoning, over zucchini**
3. **Cook on grill until brown 3 to 4 minutes per side.**
4. **Brush balsamic vinegar over zucchini**
5. **Cook 1 minute more**

Serves 2

BEEF 'n VEGETABLE STIR FRY

1 cup uncooked Basmati rice

1 cup water

1 lb. grass fed beef

1 onion sliced

2.5 cups frozen Broccoli florets thawed

1 red bell pepper cut into strips

4 tablespoons stir fry sauce (purchased)

4 tablespoons water

2 teaspoons grated ginger root (or canned spice)

1. Cook rice in 2 cups of water till tender
2. In Medium nonstick skillet, cook grass fed beef and onion over medium heat until beef is thoroughly cooked, stirring frequently. Drain.
3. Add all remaining ingredients; cover and cook 4 to 6 minutes until vegetables are crisp-tender, stirringly occasionally, serve vegetable mixture over rice.
4. Serves 4

Dietary fiber 3 g, Protein 17g, Vitamin A 25%, Calcium 2%, Vitamin C 70%, Iron 20%

BEEFY STUFFED ZUCCHINI

3 Zucchini, sliced in half lengthwise

2 teaspoons canola oil

1 lb. grass fed beef

½ chopped onion

½ cup chopped red bell pepper

1 tablespoon grated Parmesan cheese

½ teaspoon dried basil

½ teaspoon dried oregano

¼ teaspoon black pepper

½ cup no-salt added tomato sauce

¼ cup shredded reduced-fat mozzarella cheese

1. Preheat oven to 400 degree. Coat a baking sheet with cooking spray. With a spoon, scoop meat out of zucchini halves; set aside shell and chop zucchini meat finely.
2. In a medium –sized skillet, heat oil over medium –high heat and sauté ground beef, onion and red bell pepper for 6-8 minutes or until beef is no longer pink. Stir in chopped zucchini, Parmesan cheese, basil oregano, black pepper, and 1/3 cup tomato saute, and cook for 3-5 minutes, or until tender.
3. Stuff zucchini shells evenly with meat mixture, spoon remaining tomato sauce evenly over zucchini, and place on baking sheet. Cover with foil and bake for 30 minutes.

4. Remove foil and top evenly with mozzarella cheese. Bake 5-10 minutes more, or until zucchini are tender and cheese is melted.

Serves 6

BLACK BEAN AND SAUSAGE SOUP

4 oz. Kielbasa sausage

1 medium onion cut into 1inch pieces

2 cloves of garlic

2 (15 oz. cans) Black Beans drained

1 (14 oz. can) ready to serve beef broth (low sodium)

1 teaspoon cumin

½ teaspoon hot pepper sauce

2 tablespoons chopped fresh parsley

Instructions:

1. In food processor bowl with metal blade or blender container.
2. Process sausage till coarsely chopped.
3. Transfer to medium sauce pan.
4. Add onion and garlic to saucepan.
5. Add onion and garlic to food processor bowl
6. Process until finely chopped.
7. Add to sausage in saucepan and cook and stir sausage. Add onion and garlic and cook over medium high heat 4 to 5 minutes or until onion is tender.
8. Place 1 cup black beans and 1'/2 cup broth in food processor bow. Process until smooth.
9. Add pureed beans, remaining beans and broth, cumin and hot pepper sauce to ingredients in saucepan; mix well.
10. Bring to a boil stirring occasionally,
11. Sprinkle individual servings with cilantro

Serves 3 1/3 cup servings

Calories 380, Protein 23g, carbohydrates 47g, Dietary fiber 16g. Calcium 8%, Iron 30%, Vitamin
C 10%, Niacin 8%,

CABBAGE, POTATO & SAUSAGE SOUP

1 lb. cooked kielbasa or polish sausage cut in half lengthwise, sliced

1 cabbage shredded

2 (14oz) package ready to serve chicken broth

3 cups water

1 teaspoon minced garlic in water from 4.5 oz. jar

¼ teaspoon salt (optional)

¼ teaspoon pepper

2 cups Hungry Jack Mashed Potato flakes

1. In a large pot combine all ingredients except mashed potato flakes; mix well. Bring to a boil over medium-high heat, stirring occasionally.

2. Reduce heat to medium- low; simmer 5 to 10 minutes or until cabbage is almost tender

3. Remove pot from heat. Stir in mashed potato flakes

6 (1 ½ cups) servings

Dietary fiber 2 g, Protein 16g, Vitamin A 45%, Calcium 8%, Vitamin C 30%, Iron 10%

CAULIFLOWER SOUP

½ onion, finely diced

1 carrot finely diced

1 celery stalk, finely diced

1 cauliflower head, cored and roughly chopped

8 cups low-sodium chicken broth or stock and water

2 teaspoons of all-purpose flour

2 cups skim milk

1 cup half-and-half

1 teaspoons salt

Ground pepper to taste

1. Add all the above ingredients in a large sauce pan except milk and half-and-half. Cook till cauliflower, onions, carrots and celery are tender; about 20 minutes.
2. Add skim milk and half-and-half with 2 tablespoons of flour to prevent curdling and helps thicken soup.

3. After blending flour with milk add to soup till hot and ready to serve.

Serves 4

CAULIFLOWER WITH SESAME TOASTED CASHEWS

1. Bring a saucepan of water to a boil
2. Add 6 cups cauliflower florets
3. Boil 6 minutes, drain
4. Heat tablespoons sesame oil in a skillet over medium heat
5. Add 1/3 cup cashew halves
6. 1 teaspoons grated fresh ginger
7. $\frac{1}{4}$ teaspoon pepper & salt
8. Cook 4 minutes
9. Toss cauliflower with nut mixture
10. Top with 2 tablespoons of green onions

Serves 6

Calories 112

CRAB BISQUE

2 cans Cream of Mushroom Soup

2 cans Asparagus soup

4 cans of milk

½ & ½ 2 cups

Imitation crab one package 12 oz.

Sherry

Heat till done.

<u>CRAB CAKE RECIPE</u>

<u>1 egg</u>

<u>3 tablespoons Mayonnaise</u>

<u>1/8 teaspoon red pepper flakes</u>

<u>4 tablespoons lemon juice</u>

<u>1 tablespoon green onions</u>

<u>Pepper</u>

<u>Stir in crab meat</u>

<u>l/2 cup crushed buttery crackers</u>

<u>Form into patties</u>

<u>Butter in skillet</u>

<u>5-6 minutes on each side</u>

<u>Sauce – Plum, Hollandaise, avocado, mustard</u>

CRAB STUFFED MUSHROOMS

1 lb. fresh mushrooms

7 oz. crabmeat

5 green onions, thinly sliced

¼ teaspoon dried thyme

¼ teaspoon dried oregano

¼ teaspoon ground black pepper

¼ cup grated Parmesan cheese

1/3 cup mayonnaise

3 tablespoons grated Parmesan cheeses

¼ teaspoon paprika

1. Preheat oven to 350F
2. In a medium bowl, combine crabmeat, green onions, herbs, and pepper. Mix in mayonnaise and ¼ cup Parmesan cheese until well combined. Refrigerate filling until ready to use.
3. Wipe the mushrooms clean with a damp towel. Remove stems. Spoon out the gills and the base of the stem, making deep cups. Discard gills and stems. Fill the mushroom caps with rounded teaspoonful of filling, and place them in an ungreased shallow baking dish. Sprinkle tops with Parmesan and paprika.

EGGPLANT PARMESAN

3 eggplants peeled and thinly sliced

2 eggs, beaten

4 cups Italian seasoned bread crumbs

6 cups spaghetti sauced, divided

1 (16 oz.) package mozzarella cheese, shredded and divided

½ cup grated Parmesan cheese, divided

½ teaspoon dried basis

1. Preheat oven to 350 degrees
2. Dip eggplant in egg, then in bread crumbs. Place in a single layer on a baking sheet. Bake in a preheated oven for 5 minutes on each side.
3. In a 9x13 inch baking dish spread spaghetti sauce to cover the bottom. Place a layer of eggplant slices in the sauce.
4. Sprinkle with mozzarella and Parmesan cheeses. Repeat with remaining ingredients, ending with the cheeses.
5. Sprinkle basil on top.
6. Bake in preheated oven for 35 minutes, or until golden brown.

Serves 4

FESTIVE PEPPER AND ZUCCHINI STIR FRY

2 sweet peppers

2 yellow peppers

2 sweet green peppers

2-3 small zucchini

$\frac{1}{4}$ c. olive oil

1-2 clove fresh garlic

Salt & pepper

Parmesan cheese (optional)

1. Wash and clean out peppers and cut into narrow strips. Wash and trim zucchini and slice also into narrow strips.

2. Heat oil and sauté zucchini for 4-5 minutes until lightly browned. Stir in the garlic, cook 1 minute, and then add the peppers. Continues Sautéing till you reach the desired texture.

3. Turn off heat adding cheese if desired

Serves 4

HARVEST RATATOUILLE

2 tablespoons olive oil or vegetable oil

1 small red or green pepper, coarsely chopped

½ cup chopped onion

1 garlic clove minced

1 ½ cups diced eggplant

1 cup diced zucchini

1 cup diced yellow summer squash

\1 medium tomato, chopped

1 tablespoon chopped fresh parsley

1 teaspoon chopped fresh oregano

1 teaspoon chopped fresh dill weed

Pepper

2 tablespoons grated Parmesan cheese

1. Heat oil in medium skillet or wok over medium high heat until hot. Add bell pepper, onion and garlic: cook and stir 2 – 3 minutes or until crisp-tender.
2. Stir in eggplant, zucchini and summer squash; cook and stir 5 – 7 minutes or until crisp – tender.
3. Stir in all remaining ingredients except Parmesan cheese; cook until thoroughly heated. Sprinkle with Parmesan cheese.

2 (1 3/4cup) Servings

Total carbohydrates – 17 g

Dietary fiber 6 g

Protein – 6 g

Vitamin A 45%, calcium 10%, Vitamin C 90%, Iron 8%

ITALIAN MUSHROOM SOUP

1 teaspoon Olive Oil

½ cup finely chopped onion

¼ cup chopped fresh Parsley

2 garlic cloves, minced

2 lb. fresh mushrroms sliced (assorted)

2 (14 ½ oz) cans chicken broth with less sodium

½ cup of sour cream (non-fat if preferred)

1.In large sauce heat oil over medium heat until hot. Add onion, parsley, and garlic; cook and stir 2 minutes or until onion is tender

2. Add mushrooms and broth. Bring to a boil over medium-high heat. Cook and stir 4 minutes. Reduce heat to low; simmer 10 minutes

3. Stir in sour cream. Serve immediately

Makes 4 (1 ½ cup) servings

Total fat 2 g

Total carbohydrates 17 g

Dietary fiber 3 g

Protein 10 g

Vitamin A 8%, calcium 6%, vitamin C 15%, Iron 15%

LEFTOVER PORK TENDERLOIN STIR FRY

Leftover Pork tenderloin – cubed – (Put in skillet last to warm only)

1 Pepper any color – diced

1 Small Onion – diced

1 Fresh broccoli – cut stems off to make flowerets'

1 cup Basmati Rice cooked

Soy sauce – To Taste

Sweet & sour sauce -1/4 cup

Put all ingredients in a skillet with canola oil or butter. Stir Fry till all ingredients are tender. Put over Basmati rice & serve.

LOW CARB ZUCCHINI FRIES

2 Zucchini

1 tablespoon salt

2 eggs

½ cup ground almonds

½ cup grated Parmesan cheese

½ teaspoon dried Italian herb seasoning

1. Preheat oven to 425 degrees. Line a baking sheet with parchment paper.
2. Cut Zucchini into 3inch lengths, then but each piece into 9 fries. Place zucchini into a colander and sprinkle with salt. Let the zucchini pieces drain for at least I hour to remove excess liquid.
3. Beat eggs in a shallow bowl. Mix almonds, Parmesan cheese, and Italian seasoning in a second shallow bowl. Rinse salt off zucchini and pat dry with paper towels.
4. Dip each zucchini piece into beaten egg and roll in almond coating. Place coated dries on prepared baking sheet.
5. Bake in the preheated oven until the zucchini are tender and coating is crisp and browned, about 25 minutes turning them halfway through cooking time.

Serves 4 (serve warm)

LOWER-FAT, LOWER CARB POTATO CAULIFLOWER MASH

1. 1 lb. chopped peeled baking potato
2. 1 lb. cauliflower florets
3. ½ cup warm 2% milk
4. 2 tablespoons butter
5. ½ teaspoon salt (optional)
6. ¼ teaspoon black pepper

1. Boil 1 pound chopped peeled baked potato 15 minutes or until tender
2. Drain, mash
3. Coat 1pound cauliflower florets with cooking spray
4. Roast at 400degrees for 15 minutes or until browned
5. Place cauliflower in a food processor, process until smooth.
6. Fold cauliflower into potatoes
7. Add ½ cup warm 2% milk, 2 tablespoons butter salt, and ¼ teaspoon of pepper
8. Stir well

Serves 6

Calories 122

MEATLESS JAMBALAYA

1 tablespoon oil

½ cup coarsely chopped onion

12 cup chopped green bell pepper

2 garlic cloves minced

2 cups water

1 (14-5-oz) can stewed tomatoes, undrained cut up

1 (8oz) can tomato sauce

½ teaspoon dried Italian seasoning

¼ teaspoon ground red pepper

1/8 teaspoon fennel seed, crushed

1 cup uncooked basmati long grain rice

1 (15.5-oz) can butter beans, drained and rinses

1 (15.5-oz) can red kidney beans, drain, rinsed

1. Heat oil in large skillet over medium-high heat until hot. Add onion, bell pepper & garlic. Cook & stir 2 – 3 minutes or until crisp-tender.
2. Stir in water, tomatoes, tomato sauce, Italian seasoning, ground red pepper & fennel. Bring to a boil, add rice. Reduce heat to low, cover & simmer 25 to 35 minutes or until rice is tender, stirring occasionally.
3. 3. Stir in beans. Cover; simmer an additional 5 to 10 minutes or until thoroughly heated, stirring occasionally.

Calories 260 –l l/4 cups

Carbohydrates 52 g

Dietary fiber 7 g

Vitamin A 15%, Vitamin C 25 %, Calcium 8 %, iron 20%

MEXICAN BEAN SALAD

<u>Ingredients</u>

1 15 oz can black beans, drained and rinsed

1 15 oz can kidney beans, drained and rinsed

1 15 oz can chick peas, drained and rinsed

NOTE: Any Beans will do. Cannellini are great as well

1 green pepper, chopped

1 red bell pepper, chopped

1 small red onion, chopped

¼ cup olive oil (optional   I don't use it. Doesn't need it)

¼ cup red wine vinegar

1 Tbsp lemon juice

1 tsp sea salt

2-4 cloves crushed garlic

¼ cup chopped fresh parsley or cilantro

2 Tsp cumin

2 tsp ground black pepper

1 tsp chili powder

1 dash hot pepper sauce (optional for extra heat)

In a large bowl, combine beans, chopped peppers, chopped onion.

In a smaller bowl, whisk together olive oil, red wine vinegar, lemon juice, salt, garlic, parsley, cumin,

black pepper, and chili powder and hot sauce if used. Pour dressing over the beans mix and blend well.

Chill thoroughly and serve cold.

MOROCCAN LENTIL STEW

1 cup dried lentils

1 (1lb) butternut squash, peeled; cut into ¾ inch cubes

8 small new red potatoes cut into ¾ inch cubes

1 medium onion, chopped

1 (28oz) can crushed tomatoes undrained

3 teaspoons curry powder

2 cups water

1 (8oz) pkg fresh frozen green beans thawed

In a 3 – 4-quart crock pot slower cooker, combine all ingredients except green beans; stir gently to mix. Cover: cook on low setting for 8 – 10 hours or on high for 5 to 6 hours or until lentils and potatoes are tender

During the last 15 minutes of cooking time, increase setting to high. Stir in green beans; cook additional 10 to 15 minutes or until beans are tender.

Makes 6 (1 ½ cup) servings

Saturated fat 0 g

Cholesterol 0 g

Sodium

Total carbohydrates 53 g

Dietary fiber 15 g

Sugars 8 g

Protein 13 g

Vitamin A 120%

Calcium 10%

Vitamin C 50%, Iron 30%

PEACH GOAT CHEESE SALAD WITH

LEMON POPPY SEED DRESSING

DRESSING:

2 tablespoons fresh lemon juice

¼ teaspoon Dijon Mustard

¼ teaspoon honey

Salt

¼ teaspoon black pepper

1 ½ teaspoons poppy seeds

SALAD:

4 cups mixed greens

1 Organic yellow peach, pit removed and sliced thinly

16 pecan pieces

2 oz. goat cheese, crumbled

Prepare the salad: Divide the mixed greens, peach slices, pecans and goat cheese between 2 salad

plated.

Drizzle on the dressing and serve. 2 servings

ROASTED GARLIC GRILLED VEGETABLES

<u>Ingredients</u>

1 ear of corn cut into chunks

1 medium onion cut into wedges

1 small green bell pepper, cut into chunks

1 small red bell pepper, cut into chunks

1 small yellow bell pepper, cut into chunks

1 small yellow squash, sliced

1 cup of fresh mushrooms halved

2 tablespoons oil

1 tablespoon McCormick Grill Mates Roasted garlic & Herb seasoning or your own seasonings

<u>Directions:</u>

1. Toss vegetables with oil and seasoning in large bowl
2. Place vegetables in grill basket, grill rack or thread onto skewers
3. Grill over medium heat for 12 to 15 minutes or until vegetables are tender, turning occasionally.

Serves 8

ROASTED ROOT VEGETABLE SOUP

3 Carrots cut into 1-inch pieces

1 small (about 1 lb.) butternut squash, peeled and seeded cut into 1 1/4-inch pieces

1 small (about 8 oz.) sweet potato, peeled and cut into 1 ¼- inch pieces

1 small sweet or yellow onion, peeled and cut into 1 ¼-inch pieces

2 tablespoons olive oil

Sale & Pepper to taste

5 cups homemade chicken or vegetable broth (store bought)

1. Preheat the oven for 400 degrees
2. On two foil-lined, rimmed baking sheets, combine the carrots, squash, sweet potato, and onion.
3. Drizzle with oil and toss to coat. Sprinkle with sale & pepper.
4. Roast for 40 to 50 minutes, or until very tender and slightly charred, tossing every 15 minutes. Set aside.
5. Bring the broth to a boil and reduce heat to a simmer.
6. Transfer the vegetable to a food processor and add 3 cups of the warmed broth. Blend until smooth, adding more the broth to achieve the desired consistency.
7. You may need to do this step in batches or transfer the mixture to a large bowl before adding all the broth.

Serves 6

Calories 100 per serving,

Carbohydrates 12g.

Dietary fiber 3g.

Calcium 40 mg.

<u>SHRIMP & LOBSTER LOUIS SALAD</u>

4 oz. (1.5 cups) uncooked rainbow rotini (Spiral pasta)

1/3 cup mayonnaise or salad dressing

2 tablespoons chopped green onions

3 tablespoons chili sauce

1 teaspoon lemon juice

$\frac{1}{4}$ lb. fresh or frozen shelled deveined cooked medium shrimp, thawed

$\frac{1}{4}$ lb. fresh or frozen flaked cooked lobster or crabmeat, thawed

Calories – 410

Carbohydrates 23 g

Dietary fiber 1 g

Protein 27 g

Calcium 8%, Vitamin A 15%, Vitamin C 10%, iron 20%

Serves 2

SHRIMP VEGETABLE STIR-FRY

2 teaspoons oil

1 lb. shelled fresh or frozen shrimp thawed, deveined

1 medium onion sliced

1 medium green bell pepper sliced into thin strips

3 garlic cloves minced

Instructions:

1 (14oz) can diced tomatoes (Low or no salt) Heat oil in large skillet over medium high heat.

Stir fry shrimp onion, green pepper, and garlic 6-8 minutes or until shrimp turns pink & vegetables are crisp & tender. Cook and stir 2 – 3 minutes or until thoroughly heated.

4 (1 cup) servings

Calories 150

Protein 16 g, Carbohydrates 15 gm, Potassium 640 mg

SKILLET SUCCOTASH

1 teaspoon canola oil1/2 cup diced onion

½ cup diced green bell pepper

½ cup diced celery

½ teaspoon paprika

¾ cup frozen corn

¾ cup frozen lima beans

½ cup canned low-sodium diced tomatoes

1 teaspoon dried parsley flakes or fresh parsley

¼ teas poon black pepper

<u>Instructions:</u>

1. Heat oil in large skillet over medium heat. Add onion, bel pepper and celery; cook and stir 5 minutes or until onion is translucent and bell pepper and celery are crisp-tender. Stir in paprika.

2. Add corn, lima beans and tomatoes; reduce heat. Cover and simmer 20 minutes or until beans are tender. Stir in parsley and black pepper.

Makes 4 servings

Calories – 99 g

Protein 4 g

Carbohydrates 19 g

Fiber 4 g

<u>SWEET POTATO & BRUSSEL SPROUTS SKILLET</u>

About 8 Brussel sprouts thinly sliced

Butter or olive oil

½ a medium sweet potato, diced small

Balsamic vinegar

1 cup chopped mushrooms

1 clove garlic minced

2-3 chopped scallion, white & green parts

2-4 eggs (depends upon now may you want per person)

<u>Instructions</u>

1. Preheat oven to 400 degrees

2. Heat a large skillet (cast iron or regular) over medium heat. Coat /4 cup water of skillet with butter. Add Brussel sprout slices. Let them cook 2-3 minutes per side or until they become golden brown on each side. Remove from pan and set aside on a plate.

3. Add oil to pan along with sweet potato cubes. Leave them alone to get a char on one side about 5-8 minutes. Stir them and squash with balsamic vinegar. Add the garlic & mushrooms and cook for 5-10 minutes. Add ¼ cup of water in the pan and put in the oven for 10-15 minutes till the potatoes are finished cooking.

4. Remove from oven and toss the Brussel sprouts on top. Stir in the scallion and
    seasonings.

5. In a separate skillet cook eggs over easy (depending upon how many servings you need)

6. Place the potato –Brussel sprouts mixture on individual plates and serve eggs over the
    mixture.

Serves 4

SWEET POTATO CASSEROLE

4.5 cups whipped sweet potatoes

1/3 cup milk

1 cup sugar

½ tsp. vanilla

2 beaten eggs

1 cup brown sugar

1/3 cup butter

1 cup flour

1 cup chopped pecans

<u>Instructions</u>

Grease 13 x 9 casserole dish

Spread over sweet potatoes

Bake 25 minutes 350 F

Serves 4

SWEET POTATO HASH

Ingredients:

2 tbsp. of olive oil

3 sweet potatoes, diced into chunks

½ tsp. of ground pepper

2 cloves minced garlic

Green onions, sliced for garnish

Preparation:

1. Heat oil in a large pan

2. Add the potatoes, celery and onion

3. Sprinkle with some salt and Pepper.

4. Stir until all is combined

5. Cover and cook 15 minutes until the potatoes are tender

6. Turn heat on high and add the garlic, stirring to combine

7. Cook until the potatoes are browned, stirring occasionally so the potatoes do not stick.

8. Serve the potatoes topped with sliced green onions if desired.

9. Sour cream or honey can be added to top of this hash as well.

Serves 4

VEGETARIAN LASAGNA

8 to 10 lasagna noodles cooked

16 oz 2% milk fat cottage cheese

2 packages frozen spinach (thaw completely & pat dry)

1 package of sliced mozzarella cheese

Olives

Shredded carrots

Olive oil

Chopped onions

Can of sliced mushrooms

2 cans tomato sauce

Instructions

Cook lasagna noodles according to package directions

Sauté shredded carrots, onions, mushrooms, olives with olive oil in a sauce pan. Add tomato sauce. Cook till bubbly

Layer ingredients in a 13 x 9 pan. Start with cooked lasagna noodles, cottage cheese, sautéed make mixture, spinach, top with sliced mozzarella cheese. Continue layering till it fills the 13 x 9 pan. Bake at 350 F for 1 hour till bubbly. Serves 4

VEGETARIAN SUPPER DISH

Sliced zucchini

Basmati white rice

Kidney beans

Tomatoes

Onions

Shredded 2% cheddar cheese

<u>Instructions</u>

Slice zucchini, cook basmati rice will tender about 15 minutes. Stir fry zucchini, onions till tender

Add kidney beans, and chopped tomatoes Heat thoroughly. Put over cooked basmati rice with shredded

cheddar cheese.

Serves 4

CHAPTER 4

Nutrition and Beyond

AQUACULTURE

FISH FOR THE NEXT GENERATION

I found this very interesting article in the magazine "Eating Well". It was in a series of articles regarding "future of food". This article deals with how to find ways to raise seafood better, cleaner and more efficiently using Aquaculture. In Aquaculture there are 3 major ways to raise seafood that would be cleaner and more efficient for the future. I have listed and explained the 3 ways that are used below:

1. **Marine Pen** –A cage usually mode of wire or synthetic material like nylon, that corrals fish in the ocean.

    Species – Salmon, yellowtail, branzino (European sea bass).

    Benefits – New net-pen farms are sited in locations with strong currents and rocky bottoms so waste is more easily dispersed. To combat sea lice-tiny parasites that harm farmed and nearby wild salmon-fish farmers are using small fish called lump-suckers (which nibble sea lice off salmon), warm-water baths and even lasers. The result: fewer pesticides are needed. And vaccinations lower stocking densities, fish stocks bred for better disease resistance, and adding probiotics to the fisheries' diets have reduced reliance on antibiotics.

    Future outlook – integrated systems might include a marine pen stocked with salmon, surrounded by ropes of mussels and sheets of seaweed, both which can absorb excess nitrogen and phosphorous from fish feed.

2. **Tank System** – Connected tanks, typically indoors, with filtered water continuously flowing from one tank to another, also known as a recirculating aquaculture system.

Species – Sturgeon, striped bass, steelhead trout, salmon, yellowtail, turbot, Artic char, branzino and tilapia.

Benefits – Self-containment means fish cannot escape, plus pollution and habitat destruction are minimized. As much as 98% of the waste-like uneaten food pallets and fish feces-can be captured. Depending on the type of treatment system, water can be reused up to 1,000 times. Although these systems are energy-intensive, they can be located close to urban populations so the fish won't have to travel as far to our plates, offsetting some of its carbon footprint.

Future Outlook- By 2030, up to 40% of the world's aquaculture products may be grown in tanks.

3. **Pond** – A natural or man-made fresh or saltwater pond.

Species – Shrimp, tilapia, catfish, pangasius, black and striped bass, silver carp and white surgeon.

Benefits – Older ponds were designed to be open to rivers, estuaries or coastal zones for easy access to fresh water. But today's improved ponds use "closed systems" designs that prevent both pollution discharges and farm-raised species from escaping. Advances in water filtration remove waste and chemicals (like fertilizers or antibiotics), and recirculating systems allow farmers to reuse water. Adjacent treatment or settlement ponds safely keep waste out of nearby water sources.

Future outlook – Pond aquaculture had been one of the leading causes of coastal mangrove loss. Mangrove trees are important because they trap carbon and reduce flooding and erosion. Countries including Ecuador, India, Indonesia, Thailand and Vietnam have enacted stronger laws to protect them from further devastation.

As you can understand from the article regarding aquaculture, there is a lot being done to protect our seafood resources in the future for generations to come.

<u>HEALTHY TO THE BONE</u>

"Four simple strategies to shore up your skeleton and prevent osteoporosis

By Jessica Migala (Eating Well Magazine)

<u>You are never too young to start caring for bones.</u>

Through young adulthood, building bone mass is key because women's bone mineral density can begin to decline as early as age 35-and by the time you reach menopause, that loss speeds up, dipping as much as 20% over the next five years to seven years. Men's bone loss trends to start later, but that doesn't make it any less serious. (In fact the average man's risk of osteoporosis related fracture after the age of 50 is greater than his risk of prostate cancer.) For both men and women, the sooner you take steps to slow that process and maintain the bone mass you have now-or even increased it-the better.

<u>Pack in Protein</u>

The nutrients act as the glue in bones, holding together minerals like calcium, phosphorous and magnesium that keep them hard and strong, "says Taylor Wallace Ph.D. adjunct nutrition professor at George Mason University in Fairfax, Virginia. The best type of protein for bones-plant versus animal-has long been up for debate. However, an analysis of seven studies, which Wallace co-authored, found that they are usually good. Most important is getting enough. He recommends aiming for 0.365 grams of protein per pound of body weight and up to 0.56 gram for adults over age 50.For example, a 140-pound woman should get up to 78 grams of protein daily.to put that into perspective, 3 ounces of chicken breast contain 26 grams of protein and 1 cup of beans has about 14 grams.

Lift a Little

Strength training stimulates new bone development. Heavy lifting is still the gold standard for triggering this process, but you can get a similar benefit from doing lots of reps with light resistance, according to a study published in the Journal of Sport's Medicine and Physical Fitness. Lifting light for 3 times a week for 6 months increased bone mineral density by as much as 8%. Pick up a dumbbell that is 20% of the max weights you can lift (so 4 pounds if you are able to lift 20 lbs.) For each exercise do as many reps as possible in 5 minutes bursts over a course of an hour-long workout. "

Summary

The above article from "Eating Well" is a great quick way to increase bone mass. It is ways you can fit into your everyday life benefit you to improve your bone density whether a man or woman. It not only helps you build more bone mass but it is part of a healthy lifestyle.

KITCHEN OF THE FUTURE

I found a very interesting article in Eating Well Magazine called "Kitchen of The Future". I normally would pass it off as something in the distant future not worth reading but curiosity got the better of me. I began to read the article and thought it would be of great interest to us all so I decided to share it with you my readers.

1. <u>At-Home Water-from-Air Generator</u>. As regions in the West and Southwest become drier, water rationing could make "DIY water "solutions essential kitchen gear. The Watergren "Genny" device (not yet available) scours indoor air for available moisture and turns it into drinkable water.

2. <u>Compact "Turbo" Oven -</u> Powerful, portable countertop oven could replace built-in-units in many kitchens, especially urban ones. The Brava oven hints at what are possible-aiming high-intensity light rays to simultaneously cook different foods at different temperatures, and cutting cooking times buy half or more.

3. <u>Electric Tea Kettle</u> –The National Renewable Energy Laboratory predicts that by 2050 as fossil fuels fun out, electricity will up to 94% of all home cooking. By then, most Americans will have discovered the European-style speed and efficiency of boiling water in a plug-in countertop kettle.

4. <u>Facial Recognition Smart Pet Bowl</u> – In 2018 Americans spend $72 billion on pets and the number is rising. The trends has fueled everything from pet-food delivery services to tech like the Mookkie smart pet food dispenser, due out later this year, which uses facial recognition to make sure that pets eat only their own kibble. (I can relate).

5. <u>Composting Device</u> – Small electric composters Like the Zera Food Recycler could be a mainstay of kitchens, drastically reducing waste by churning food scraps-including meat and dairy-into house-plant ready compost overnight.

6. <u>Kitchen "Co-bot"</u> – By 2030, robots like Samsung's Bot Chef, will chop, mix, lift and pour in many homes, a game-changer for the 61% of older adults who want to age at home but will need help with the physical demands of cooking.

7. <u>Countertop Dishwasher</u> – As the numbers of untethered apartment dwellers, singles and seniors in Europe grow, a "BYO appliance" trend is taking off. By 2030, devices like Heatworks Tetra countertop; (and portable) dishwasher will be common the U.S. too.

8. <u>RF Oven</u> – Full-size ovens will be automated, connected, multifunctional and fast. Miele's new Dialog is the first consumer appliance to employ radio frequency (RF) technology, using electromagnetic waves to cook food precisely and up to 70% faster. Electric heating elements ensure professional results when baking and roasting.

9. <u>Multitasking Water Faucet</u> – By 2030, specialty faucets (like Zip Water's new HydroTap Celsius All-in-one) will provide chilled, boiling and carbonated water-even milk or coffee- on demand. Concerns about municipal water supplies will lead to adoption of advanced filtration systems that include toxin sensing.

10. <u>Personal Pots and Pans</u> – Today, some 28% of American households are just one person, up from 13% in the 1960's. This demographic is expected to continue growing and manufacturers will respond with offerings ranging from mini appliances and food portions to personal-size grill pans and Dutch ovens.

11. <u>Kitchen Island</u> - As lines between kitchen and living room continue to blur, the island will remain at the center, surrounded by "lounge-y" couches, coffee tables and even carpeted floors. Adding to the ambiance, finishes that mimic timber or stone will allow appliance to blend into the living space seamlessly.

I can see myself using some of the items in the above article especially as we age.

BIBLIOGRAPHY

Alderman H, Michael, McCarron, A. David, "Are you getting too much salt in your diet, Probably Not",

Wall Street Journal, June 2019

Bluestein, Adam. "The Kitchen of Tomorrow", Eating Well October 2019

Jung, Carolyn, "Fish for the Next Generation, Aquaculture", Eating Well, October 2019

Peters, Sally, Publisher, Fast and Healthy Glossary, 1998 pp. 12-14

Heaner, Martica PhD, "Good News for Carb Lovers" Consumer Reports, November 2017

Megala, Jessica, "Healthy to the Bone", Eating Well, Jan 2017

Mitchell, Heidi, "How Much Protein Should Eat Each Day? Wall Street Journal, July 2019

<u>ABOUT THE AUTHOR</u>

I was born & raised in Cleveland Ohio and later moved to Akron, Ohio. My husband & I moved to North Carolina in 2014 where we currently live with our two cats, Bonnie & Clyde.

I am a sibling of 3 other family members one of whom is my fraternal twin sister. My father was a doctor who started out in obstetrics and later internal medicine. My mother was a Registered Nurse who was my father's nurse in his office for years. This was how I began to be interested in well-being and nutrition. I can remember when we were about 13 years old and my father decided that our lunches, we took to school needed to be healthier. He substituted pies, cakes cookies for fruit and other healthy foods. Even though it seemed mean at the time I realize now how it benefited me later in life.

My mother, in addition to being a fabulous mother, was a terrific cook. She would prepare the healthiest meals but also were delicious but nutritious.

My parents were advocates of getting plenty of exercise early in my life. In our early teens my sister & I rode hunter-jumper horses and showed them in several states. That kept us very busy. I also participated in various other sports such as tennis, volley bowl, swimming and walking. To this day I walk 2 miles every morning summer and winter. I also lift light weights daily for strengthening exercises.

Before moving to North Carolina, I worked at Kaiser Permanente in Ohio as a Medical Records Technician. I started my job fairly early in the morning so I would bring a change of clothes to work and go out at noon on my lunch hour to get 2 miles of walking in every day. My boss

would let me use the closet in our room to change with a sign on it "occupied". You know the

winters in Ohio could be very brutal but I would go out every day even in the very cold weather

to exercise, rain or snow. I even would have some of my co-workers join me during nice

weather.

After almost 20 years in the Medical Record field, it became apparent from reading and coding

the charts that the following stagnant lifestyles contributed to poor health. I saw the diagnoses

of diabetes, obesity, hyperlipidemia (high cholesterol) hypertension so much on the charts that

I had the diagnoses codes for those diseases memorized. I soon realized that almost 60% of

Americans are overweight? It is time for a change to a healthier lifestyle!